FATTY LIVER DIET COOKBOOK FOR WOMEN

The

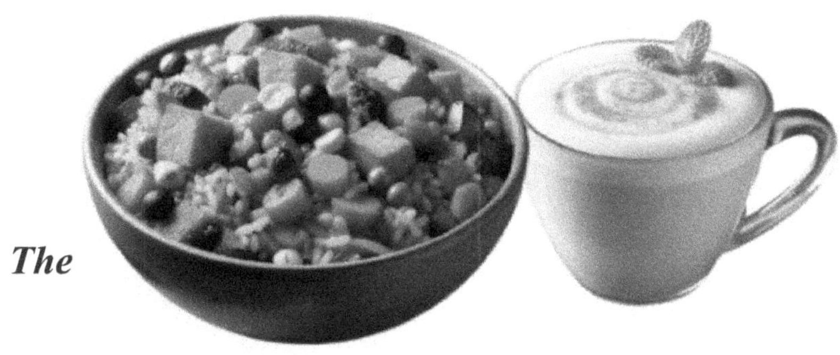

Ultimate Guide to Managing Fatty Liver Disease with Simple and Nutritious Meals

Lanita Cruz

Copyright © 2024 by Lanita Cruz

TABLE OF CONTENT

Disclaimer

The information provided in this cookbook is for educational and informational purposes only. It is not intended to be a substitute for professional medical advice, diagnosis, or treatment.

Always seek the advice of your physician or other qualified health provider with any questions you may have regarding a medical condition.

The recipes and dietary suggestions included are based on general principles and may not be suitable for everyone.

Individual dietary needs and health conditions vary, and it is essential to consult with a healthcare professional before making significant changes to your diet.

The author and publisher disclaim responsibility for any effects resulting directly or indirectly from the use or misuse of the information provided in this cookbook.

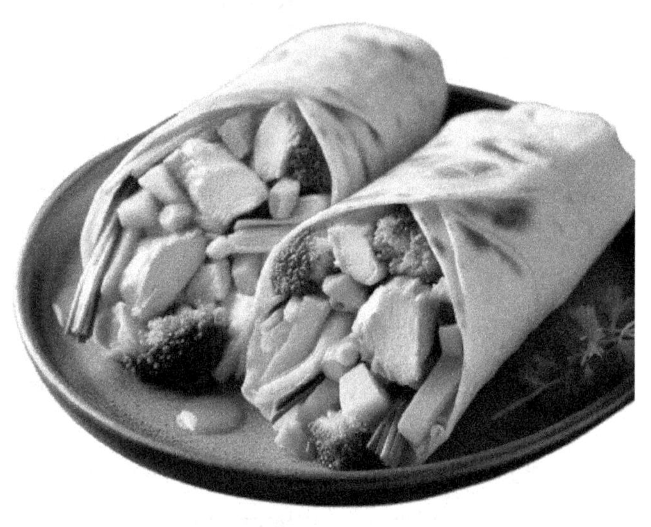

Introduction

Are you tired of feeling weighed down by fatigue and discomfort? Do you find yourself longing for the vitality and energy you once had?

Perhaps you've been on a journey to reclaim your health, but haven't found the right path yet – **"Fatty Liver Diet Cookbook for Women"** is the perfect path!

Picture this: waking up every morning with a spring in your step, feeling light and vibrant throughout the day, and enjoying delicious meals that not only tantalize your taste buds but also nourish your body internally.

Sounds like a dream, doesn't it? Well, let me assure you, it's entirely within your reach.

Fatty liver disease is a common and often silent condition that affects millions of people around the world. It occurs when excess fat accumulates in your liver cells, causing inflammation and damage.

If left untreated, fatty liver disease can lead to serious complications, such as cirrhosis, liver cancer, and liver failure.

You may be wondering: how did I get fatty liver disease? How can I reverse it and prevent it from getting worse? What can I eat and what should I avoid? How can I improve my liver health and overall well-being?

These are some of the questions that you may have, and that this book will answer for you.

In this book, you'll discover the principles of the fatty liver diet, a dietary approach that can help you heal your liver and restore its function.

You will learn the benefits of the fatty liver diet, the foods to eat and avoid, and how to plan your meals and snacks.

You will also find a comprehensive shopping list for the fatty liver diet, to make your grocery shopping easier and more convenient. You will also discover the keys to unlocking a healthier, happier you.

But before we go into the specifics, let's set the stage for what lies ahead.

What do you expect to gain from this journey? Is it a deeper understanding of nutrition and its impact on your body?

Are you seeking easy and practical guidance on how to make sustainable lifestyle changes because of your health? Or perhaps you're simply on a journey to avoid having a fatty liver?

Whatever your goals may be, rest assured that this book is not just another addition to the sea of diet and health guides. It's a personalized roadmap crafted with your healing in mind.

Unlike other books that overwhelm you with complex theories and rigid rules, this one is designed to empower you with practical knowledge and delicious recipes tailored specifically for women and anyone dealing with fatty liver issues or trying to avoid fatty liver issues.

You're not alone in this journey. Thousands, if not millions, of women around the world are facing similar struggles.

Yet, with the right support and guidance, each one has the potential to rewrite their health story. And that's precisely what I aim to do with this book.

So, if you're ready to take charge of your health and embark on this delicious and healing journey, turn the page and let's begin. Let's make every moment count. Are you ready?

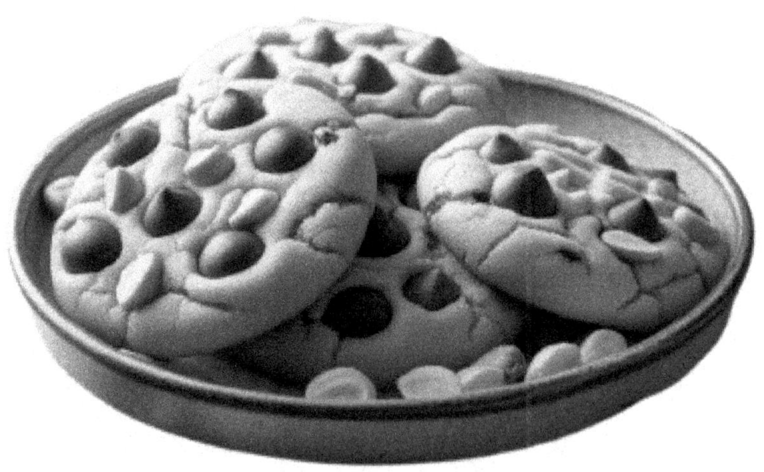

CHAPTER 1

Principles of the Fatty Liver Diet

1. **Balanced Nutrition:** Your journey begins with nourishing your body with a balanced array of whole foods.

   Think colorful fruits, crisp vegetables, lean proteins, and hearty whole grains. These nutrient-packed options fuel your body while supporting your liver's functions.

2. **Moderation and Portion Control:** It's essential to maintain balance and keep an eye on portion sizes. Practice moderation in your food choices to prevent excessive calorie intake, aiding in weight management and liver health.

3. **Limiting Added Sugars and Refined Carbs:** Keep a close watch on added sugars and refined carbohydrates lurking in processed foods.

   Opt for whole, unprocessed alternatives to stabilize blood sugar levels and reduce the risk of insulin resistance.

4. **Healthy Fats:** Embrace the right kinds of fats, such as those found in avocados, nuts, seeds, and fatty fish.

   These healthy fats support liver function and overall well-being, so don't shy away from incorporating them into your diet.

5. **Stay Hydrated:** Hydration is key for optimal liver function and detoxification. Make sure to drink plenty of water throughout the day to keep your body hydrated and your liver happy.

6. **Move Your Body:** Regular physical activity is not only beneficial for maintaining a healthy weight but also supports liver health.

   Find activities you enjoy, whether it's a brisk walk, yoga, or dancing, and make movement a part of your daily routine.

7. **Watch Your Alcohol Intake**: If you're dealing with fatty liver disease, it's crucial to limit or avoid alcohol consumption.

   Alcohol can exacerbate liver damage and hinder your body's ability to metabolize fats effectively.

By incorporating these principles into your lifestyle, you'll create an environment that nurtures your liver health and overall well-being. It's time to take charge of your health and embark on a journey toward a happier, healthier you.

Benefits of Fatty Liver Diet

1. **Improved Liver Function:** By following the Fatty Liver Diet, you can support your liver in reducing fat accumulation and improving its overall function. This leads to enhanced detoxification processes and better metabolic regulation.

2. **Weight Management:** The focus on whole foods and portion control in the Fatty Liver Diet can help you achieve and maintain a healthy weight. This is crucial for reducing the risk of fatty liver disease progression and related complications.

3. **Stabilized Blood Sugar Levels:** By limiting added sugars and refined carbohydrates, the Fatty Liver Diet helps stabilize blood sugar levels, reducing the risk of insulin resistance and type 2 diabetes.

4. **Increased Energy Levels:** Nourishing your body with nutrient-dense foods and staying hydrated can boost your energy levels and reduce feelings of fatigue and lethargy.

5. **Enhanced Digestive Health:** The Fatty Liver Diet emphasizes fiber-rich foods like fruits, vegetables, and whole grains, which promote healthy digestion and regular bowel movements.

6. **Reduced Inflammation:** Many foods included in the Fatty Liver Diet, such as fruits, vegetables, and omega-3 fatty acids, have anti-inflammatory properties.

   By incorporating these foods into your diet, you can help reduce inflammation in the body, which is beneficial for overall health.

7. **Lower Risk of Chronic Diseases:** Following the Fatty Liver Diet not only improves liver health but also reduces the risk of developing other chronic diseases such as cardiovascular disease, hypertension, and certain types of cancer.

By embracing the Fatty Liver Diet, you can experience a wide range of health benefits that will not only improve your liver health but also enhance your overall well-being and quality of life.

Foods to Eat

Fruits: Fill your basket with a colorful assortment of fruits like apples, berries, oranges, and grapes. These juicy delights are not only packed with vitamins and antioxidants but also provide natural sweetness to satisfy your cravings.

Vegetables: Load up on nutrient-rich veggies such as spinach, kale, broccoli, and bell peppers.

These powerhouse greens are low in calories and high in fiber, making them perfect for supporting liver health and keeping you feeling full and satisfied.

Whole Grains: Swap out refined grains for whole grains like quinoa, brown rice, oats, and barley. These wholesome grains are rich in fiber and essential nutrients, providing sustained energy and supporting digestive health.

Lean Proteins: Choose lean sources of protein such as skinless poultry, tofu, fish, and legumes.

These protein-packed options are vital for muscle repair and growth, as well as for keeping you feeling full and satiated.

Healthy Fats: Don't shy away from fats! Opt for sources of healthy fats like avocados, seeds, nuts, and olive oil. These fats provide essential fatty acids that support brain health, reduce inflammation, and promote overall well-being.

Dairy or Dairy Alternatives: Incorporate low-fat dairy products or dairy alternatives like almond milk or soy yogurt into your diet. These options provide calcium and vitamin D for strong bones and teeth, without the excess saturated fat.

Herbs and Spices: Add flavor to your meals with herbs and spices like garlic, ginger, turmeric, and cinnamon.

Not only do these aromatic additions enhance the taste of your dishes, but they also offer a range of health benefits, including anti-inflammatory properties.

Foods to Avoid

Added Sugars: Say goodbye to sugary treats like candy, soda, and baked goods. These sweet temptations can wreak havoc on your liver and spike your blood sugar levels, leading to inflammation and weight gain.

Refined Carbohydrates: Bid farewell to refined grains like white bread, white rice, and pasta.

These carbohydrate-heavy culprits lack fiber and essential nutrients, causing rapid spikes in blood sugar and promoting fat accumulation in the liver.

Trans Fats: Avoid foods high in trans fats, such as fried foods, commercially baked goods, and packaged snacks.

These artery-clogging fats not only contribute to liver fat accumulation but also increase the risk of heart disease and other chronic conditions.

Highly Processed Foods: Cut back on highly processed foods like fast food, microwave meals, and processed meats.

These convenient but nutritionally devoid options are packed with unhealthy fats, sugars, and additives that can wreak havoc on your liver and overall health.

Excessive Alcohol: Limit or eliminate alcohol consumption, as it can contribute to liver damage and exacerbate fatty liver disease.

Even moderate alcohol intake can strain your liver's ability to metabolize fats and toxins, leading to inflammation and liver damage over time.

Sugary Beverages: Ditch sugary drinks like fruit juices, sweetened teas, and energy drinks. These liquid calories provide little to no nutritional value and can contribute to weight gain and liver fat accumulation.

High-Sodium Foods: Cut back on foods high in sodium, such as processed meats, canned soups, and salty snacks.

Excessive sodium intake can lead to fluid retention and liver inflammation, so opt for fresh, whole foods whenever possible.

Comprehensive Shopping List for Fatty Liver Diet

Fresh Fruits:

- Apples

- Berries (strawberries, blueberries, raspberries)
- Oranges
- Bananas
- Pears
- Kiwi
- Grapefruit
- Cherries

Fresh Vegetables:

- Spinach
- Kale
- Broccoli
- Cauliflower
- Bell peppers (red, green, yellow)
- Carrots
- Cucumbers
- Tomatoes
- Onions
- Garlic

Whole Grains:

- Quinoa

- Brown rice

- Oats

- Barley

- Whole wheat bread

- Whole wheat pasta

- Bulgur

- Millet

Lean Proteins:

- Skinless poultry (chicken breast, turkey)

- Fish (salmon, trout, tuna)

- Tofu

- Tempeh

- Eggs

- Legumes (beans, lentils, chickpeas)

Healthy Fats:

- Avocados

- Almonds

- Walnuts

- Chia seeds

- Flaxseeds

- Olive oil

- Coconut oil

Dairy or Dairy Alternatives:

- Low-fat yogurt

- Almond milk

- Soy milk

- Tofu-based cheese

- Cottage cheese

Herbs and Spices:

- Garlic

- Ginger

- Turmeric

- Cinnamon

- Basil

- Parsley

- Cilantro

- Cumin

- Paprika

Non-Starchy Vegetables:

- Leafy greens (lettuce, arugula, spinach)
- Celery
- Asparagus
- Zucchini
- Eggplant
- Mushrooms

Low-Sodium Broth:

- Vegetable or chicken broth (low-sodium varieties)

Sweeteners:

- Stevia
- Honey
- Maple syrup (in moderation)

CHAPTER 2

Breakfast Recipes for Fatty Liver Diet

Chia Seed Pudding with Berries and Coconut Flakes

- **Preparation Time:** 5 minutes (plus chilling time)
- **Serves:** 2

Ingredients:

- 1/4 cup chia seeds
- 1 cup almond milk (or any low-fat milk)
- 1 tablespoon maple syrup (optional)
- 1/2 teaspoon vanilla extract
- 1/2 cup mixed berries (such as strawberries, raspberries & blueberries)
- 2 tablespoons coconut flakes

Nutritional Information: Per serving - Calories: 215kcal | Carbohydrates: 18g | Protein: 5g | Fat: 14g | Saturated Fat: 3g | Sodium: 98mg | Potassium: 164mg | Fiber: 10g | Sugar: 5g | Vitamin C: 2mg | Calcium: 271mg | Iron: 2mg

Instructions:

1. In a bowl, combine chia seeds, almond milk, maple syrup (if using), and vanilla extract, stir well to ensure the chia seeds are evenly distributed.
2. Cover the bowl and refrigerate for at least 2 hours or overnight, allowing the chia seeds to absorb the liquid and thicken into a pudding-like consistency.
3. Once the chia pudding is ready, divide it into serving glasses or bowls.
4. Top each serving with mixed berries and coconut flakes.
5. Serve chilled and enjoy the creamy texture and burst of fruity flavors.

Serving Suggestions:

- For an extra indulgent treat, drizzle a little extra maple syrup or honey on top before serving. Add a dollop of Greek yogurt for added creaminess and protein.

Viking Crispbread with Salmon

- **Preparation Time:** 10 minutes
- **Serves:** 2

Ingredients:

- 4 pieces of whole grain crispbread
- 4 ounces smoked salmon slices
- 1/4 cup low-fat cream cheese
- 1 tablespoon capers, drained
- 1/4 red onion, thinly sliced
- Fresh dill, for garnish

Nutritional Information: Per serving - Calories: 240kcal | Carbohydrates: 22g | Protein: 16g | Fat: 10g | Saturated Fat: 4g | Cholesterol: 15mg | Sodium: 600mg | Fiber: 6g | Sugar: 2g

Instructions:

1. Spread a thin layer of low-fat cream cheese on each piece of crispbread.
2. Top the cream cheese with smoked salmon slices, dividing evenly among the crispbreads.

3. Sprinkle capers over the salmon, and add a few slices of red onion on top.

4. Garnish with fresh dill for an extra burst of flavor and aroma.

5. Serve immediately and enjoy the delicious combination of crunchy crispbread, creamy cheese, and savory smoked salmon!

Serving Suggestions:

- Pair this Viking Crispbread with Salmon with a side of fresh cucumber slices or cherry tomatoes for a refreshing and light breakfast.

Walnut or Pecan Apple Oatmeal

- **Preparation Time:** 10 minutes
- **Serves:** 2

Ingredients:

- 1 cup old-fashioned oats
- 2 cups water or milk (almond milk, soy milk, or dairy milk)
- 1 apple, cored and diced

- 1/4 teaspoon ground cinnamon

- 2 tablespoons chopped walnuts or pecans

- 1 tablespoon honey or maple syrup (if desired)

- Pinch of salt

Nutritional Information: Per serving - Calories: 250kcal | Carbohydrates: 42g | Protein: 7g | Fat: 7g | Saturated Fat: 1g | Sodium: 10mg | Fiber: 6g | Sugar: 15g | Vitamin C: 4mg | Calcium: 50mg | Iron: 2mg

Instructions:

1. In a saucepan, bring water or milk to a boil over medium heat, stir in oats, diced apple, ground cinnamon, and a pinch of salt.

2. Reduce heat to low and simmer, stirring occasionally, for about 5 minutes or until the oats are creamy and tender.

3. Once the oats are cooked, remove from heat and stir in chopped walnuts or pecans.

4. If desired, sweeten with honey or maple syrup to taste.

5. Divide the oatmeal into serving bowls and garnish with additional chopped nuts and a sprinkle of cinnamon, if desired.

6. Serve hot and enjoy the comforting warmth and delicious flavors of Walnut or Pecan Apple Oatmeal!

Serving Suggestions:

- You can customize this recipe by adding other fruits such as sliced bananas or berries for added sweetness and variety.

Blueberry and Granola Yogurt Parfait

- **Preparation Time:** 10 minutes
- **Serves:** 2

Ingredients:

- 1 cup plain Greek yogurt
- 1 cup fresh blueberries
- 1/2 cup granola (choose a low-sugar and whole grain variety)
- 2 tablespoons honey or maple syrup (if desired)

- 1/4 teaspoon vanilla extract

Nutritional Information: Per serving - Calories: 250kcal | Carbohydrates: 38g | Protein: 17g | Fat: 5g | Saturated Fat: 1g | Cholesterol: 10mg | Sodium: 90mg | Fiber: 4g | Sugar: 22g | Vitamin C: 8mg | Calcium: 200mg | Iron: 1mg

Instructions:

1. In a small bowl, mix together the Greek yogurt, honey or maple syrup (if using), and vanilla extract until well combined.

2. In serving glasses or bowls, layer the Greek yogurt mixture, fresh blueberries, and granola, repeating until you reach the top of the glass.

3. Start with a layer of Greek yogurt at the bottom of the glass, followed by a layer of blueberries, and then a layer of granola.

4. Repeat the layers until you use up all the ingredients, finishing with a final layer of Greek yogurt on top.

5. Drizzle a little honey or maple syrup over the top for extra sweetness, if desired.

6. Garnish with a few extra blueberries and a sprinkle of granola for added texture.

7. Serve immediately and enjoy the delightful combination of creamy yogurt, juicy blueberries, and crunchy granola!

Serving Suggestions:

- Pair this Blueberry and Granola Yogurt Parfait with a cup of freshly brewed coffee or herbal tea for a delightful and nutritious breakfast.

Toast with Avocado and Ricotta

- **Preparation Time:** 10 minutes
- **Serves:** 2

Ingredients:

- 2 slices whole grain bread
- 1 ripe avocado
- 1/2 cup ricotta cheese
- 1 tablespoon lemon juice
- Salt and pepper, to taste
- Red pepper flakes, for garnish (optional)

- Fresh basil leaves, for garnish (optional)

Nutritional Information: Per serving - Calories: 280kcal | Carbohydrates: 24g | Protein: 12g | Fat: 16g | Saturated Fat: 5g | Cholesterol: 25mg | Sodium: 230mg | Fiber: 8g | Sugar: 2g | Vitamin C: 10mg | Calcium: 180mg | Iron: 1mg

Instructions:

1. Toast the slices of whole grain bread until golden brown and crispy.
2. In a small bowl, mash the ripe avocado with a fork until smooth.
3. In another bowl, mix the ricotta cheese with lemon juice until well combined.
4. Spread a generous layer of mashed avocado on each slice of toasted bread.
5. Top the avocado with dollops of ricotta cheese mixture, spreading it evenly.
6. Season with salt and pepper to taste, garnish with red pepper flakes and fresh basil leaves, if desired, for an extra kick of flavor and freshness.

7. Serve immediately and enjoy the creamy texture and delicious flavors of Toast with Avocado and Ricotta,

Serving Suggestions:

- Pair this Toast with Avocado and Ricotta with a side of fresh fruit salad or sliced tomatoes for a refreshing and balanced breakfast. Enjoy this simple yet satisfying toast as a nutritious start to your day.

Cheese and Veggie Egg White Breakfast Sandwich

- **Preparation Time:** 15 minutes
- **Serves:** 2

Ingredients:

- 4 slices whole grain bread
- 4 egg whites
- 1/2 cup baby spinach leaves
- 1/2 cup sliced bell peppers
- 1/4 cup sliced mushrooms

- 1/4 cup shredded low-fat cheese (cheddar, mozzarella, or your choice)
- Salt and pepper, to taste
- Cooking spray or olive oil

Nutritional Information: Per serving - Calories: 260kcal | Carbohydrates: 31g | Protein: 19g | Fat: 6g | Saturated Fat: 2g | Cholesterol: 5mg | Sodium: 420mg | Fiber: 6g | Sugar: 5g | Vitamin A: 50% | Vitamin C: 80% | Calcium: 20% | Iron: 10%

Instructions:

1. Heat a non-stick skillet over medium heat and lightly coat it with cooking spray or olive oil.
2. Add the sliced bell peppers and mushrooms to the skillet and sauté until they are tender, about 3-4 minutes, season with salt and pepper to your preferred taste.
3. In a separate bowl, whisk the egg whites until frothy, pour them into the skillet and cook, stirring occasionally, until they are set and scrambled.
4. While the eggs are cooking, toast the slices of whole grain bread until golden brown.

5. Once the eggs are cooked, divide them into two portions and layer them onto two slices of toasted bread.

6. Top each egg layer with baby spinach leaves and shredded cheese.

7. Place the remaining slices of toasted bread on top to create sandwiches.

8. Cut each sandwich in half diagonally and serve immediately.

Serving Suggestions:

- Customize with sliced tomatoes, avocado, or your favorite herbs and spices for extra flavor.

Cheerios and Almond Milk Bowl

- **Preparation Time:** 5 minutes
- **Serves:** 1

Ingredients:

- 1 cup Cheerios cereal (or any whole grain cereal of your choice)
- 1 cup unsweetened almond milk

- 1/2 cup fresh berries (such as strawberries, raspberries & blueberries)

- 1 tablespoon chopped nuts (such as almonds, walnuts & pecans)

- Optional: 1 tablespoon honey or maple syrup for sweetness

Nutritional Information: Per serving - Calories: 250kcal | Carbohydrates: 35g | Protein: 7g | Fat: 9g | Saturated Fat: 1g | Cholesterol: 0mg | Sodium: 220mg | Fiber: 5g | Sugar: 10g | Vitamin C: 40% | Calcium: 40% | Iron: 25%

Instructions:

1. Pour the Cheerios cereal into a bowl.
2. Add the unsweetened almond milk over the cereal.
3. Top with fresh berries and chopped nuts.
4. Drizzle with honey or maple syrup, if desired, for extra sweetness.
5. Stir gently to combine all the ingredients.
6. Enjoy immediately.

Serving Suggestions:

- Customize this recipe by adding sliced bananas, diced apples, or a sprinkle of cinnamon for extra flavor and nutrition. Enjoy this quick and easy breakfast option to start your day on a healthy note.

Lunch Recipes for Fatty Liver Diet Chicken and Vegetable Wrap with Ginger Sauce

- **Preparation Time:** 20 minutes
- **Serves:** 2

Ingredients:

- 2 large whole wheat tortillas
- 2 boneless, skinless chicken breasts, cooked and thinly sliced
- 1 cup mixed salad greens
- 1/2 cucumber, thinly sliced
- 1/2 red bell pepper, thinly sliced

- 1/4 cup shredded carrots

- 1/4 cup sliced red cabbage

- For Ginger Sauce:

- 2 tablespoons low-sodium soy sauce

- 1 tablespoon rice vinegar

- 1 tablespoon honey

- 1 teaspoon grated ginger

- 1 teaspoon sesame oil

- 1 garlic clove, minced

- Pinch of red pepper flakes (optional)

Nutritional Information: Per serving - Calories: 350kcal | Carbohydrates: 38g | Protein: 28g | Fat: 10g | Saturated Fat: 2g | Cholesterol: 60mg | Sodium: 750mg | Fiber: 6g | Sugar: 10g | Vitamin A: 120% | Vitamin C: 90% | Calcium: 15% | Iron: 20%

Instructions:

1. In a small bowl, whisk together all the ingredients for the ginger sauce until it is well combined. Set aside.

2. Lay out the whole wheat tortillas on a clean surface.

3. Place a layer of mixed salad greens in the center of each tortilla.

4. Arrange the cooked chicken slices, cucumber, red bell pepper, shredded carrots, and red cabbage on top of the greens.

5. Drizzle the prepared ginger sauce over the chicken and vegetables.

6. Fold the sides of the tortillas over the filling, then roll them tightly to form wraps.

7. Cut the wraps in half diagonally.

8. Serve immediately, and enjoy the flavorful Chicken and Vegetable Wraps with Ginger Sauce!

Serving Suggestions:

- Pair these Chicken and Vegetable Wraps with a side of oven-baked sweet potato fries or a refreshing fruit salad for a complete and satisfying lunch.

  You can also serve them with a small bowl of miso soup for an extra touch of Asian-inspired flavor

Tuna Salad Stuffed Tomato with Whole Grain Crackers

- **Preparation Time:** 15 minutes
- **Serves:** 2

Ingredients:

- 2 large ripe tomatoes
- 1 can (5 oz) tuna in water, drained
- 2 tablespoons Greek yogurt
- 1 tablespoon lemon juice
- 1/4 cup diced celery
- 2 tablespoons diced red onion
- 1 tablespoon chopped fresh parsley
- Salt and pepper, to taste
- Whole grain crackers, for serving

Nutritional Information: Per serving - Calories: 180kcal | Carbohydrates: 10g | Protein: 20g | Fat: 6g | Saturated Fat: 1g | Cholesterol: 30mg | Sodium: 270mg | Fiber: 3g | Sugar: 5g | Vitamin A: 50% | Vitamin C: 40% | Calcium: 10% | Iron: 15%

Instructions:

1. Slice off the tops of the tomatoes and carefully scoop out the seeds and pulp using a spoon to create tomato cups. Set aside.
2. In a mixing bowl, combine the drained tuna, Greek yogurt, lemon juice, diced celery, diced red onion, and chopped fresh parsley. Mix well to combine.
3. Season the tuna salad mixture with salt and pepper to taste.
4. Spoon the tuna salad mixture into the hollowed-out tomatoes, dividing it evenly between them.
5. Serve the stuffed tomatoes alongside whole grain crackers.

Serving Suggestions:

- Pair a side of mixed greens tossed in a light vinaigrette dressing for a refreshing and balanced meal. Enjoy the combination of savory tuna salad and juicy tomatoes for a satisfying lunch.

Sweet Potato and Black Bean Tacos

- **Preparation Time:** 25 minutes
- **Serves:** 2

Ingredients:

- 2 medium sweet potatoes, peeled and diced
- 1 tablespoon olive oil
- 1 teaspoon chili powder
- 1/2 teaspoon ground cumin
- 1/2 teaspoon paprika
- Salt and pepper, to taste
- 15 oz. (1 can) black beans, thoroughly drained & rinsed
- 1/2 cup diced red onion
- 1/2 cup diced bell peppers (any color)
- 1/4 cup chopped fresh cilantro
- 4 small whole wheat or corn tortillas
- Optional toppings: diced avocado, salsa, Greek yogurt or sour cream, lime wedges

Nutritional Information: Per serving (2 tacos) - Calories: 380kcal | Carbohydrates: 70g | Protein: 12g | Fat: 8g |

Saturated Fat: 1g | Cholesterol: 0mg | Sodium: 580mg | Fiber: 15g | Sugar: 10g | Vitamin A: 430% | Vitamin C: 90% | Calcium: 15% | Iron: 25%

Instructions:

1. Preheat the oven to 400°F (200°C).
2. In a large bowl, toss the diced sweet potatoes with olive oil, chili powder, cumin, paprika, salt, and pepper until evenly coated.
3. Spread the seasoned sweet potatoes in a single layer on a baking sheet lined with parchment paper.
4. Roast in the preheated oven for 20-25 minutes, or until the sweet potatoes are tender and lightly browned, stirring halfway through.
5. In the meantime, in a small saucepan, heat the black beans over medium heat until heated through.
6. Warm the tortillas in a dry skillet or in the microwave.
7. Assemble the tacos by layering the roasted sweet potatoes, black beans, diced red onion, diced bell peppers, and chopped fresh cilantro on the warmed tortillas.

8. Serve the tacos with optional toppings such as diced avocado, salsa, Greek yogurt or sour cream, and lime wedges on the side.

Serving Suggestions:

- Pair with a side of Mexican-style rice or a crisp green salad for a complete and satisfying meal. Enjoy the combination of flavorful roasted sweet potatoes and hearty black beans wrapped in warm tortillas for a delicious lunch option.

Mushroom and Spinach Quesadillas

- **Preparation Time:** 20 minutes
- **Serves:** 2

Ingredients:

- 4 large whole wheat or corn tortillas
- 2 cups sliced mushrooms (any variety)
- 2 cups fresh baby spinach leaves
- 1/2 cup diced red onion
- 1 cup of grated cheese (either Monterey Jack or a mix of Mexican cheeses)

- 1 tablespoon olive oil

- Salt and pepper, to taste

- Optional toppings: salsa, guacamole, Greek yogurt or sour cream

Nutritional Information: Per serving (1 quesadilla) - Calories: 380kcal | Carbohydrates: 40g | Protein: 15g | Fat: 18g | Saturated Fat: 8g | Cholesterol: 35mg | Sodium: 570mg | Fiber: 7g | Sugar: 5g | Vitamin A: 100% | Vitamin C: 20% | Calcium: 35% | Iron: 15%

Instructions:

1. Heat olive oil in a large skillet over medium heat, add the sliced mushrooms and diced red onion to the skillet.

2. Cook, stirring occasionally, until the mushrooms are tender and the onions are translucent, about 5-7 minutes, season with salt and pepper to taste.

3. Add the fresh baby spinach leaves to the skillet and cook until wilted, about 2-3 minutes. Remove from heat and set aside.

4. Place a tortilla on a flat surface, sprinkle a quarter of the shredded cheese evenly over one half of the tortilla.

5. Spoon a quarter of the mushroom, spinach, and onion mixture over the cheese.

6. Fold the other half of the tortilla over the filling to create a half-moon shape.

7. Repeat with the remaining tortillas and filling ingredients.

8. Heat a clean skillet or griddle over medium heat. Carefully transfer the assembled quesadillas to the skillet or griddle.

9. Cook each quesadilla for 2-3 minutes on each side, or until golden brown and the cheese is melted, remove from heat and let cool for a minute before slicing into wedges.

10. Serve the Mushroom and Spinach Quesadillas with optional toppings such as salsa, guacamole, Greek yogurt, or sour cream.

Serving Suggestions:

- Pair these Mushroom and Spinach Quesadillas with a side of Mexican-style rice or a crisp green salad for a complete and satisfying meal.

Detox Roasted Pumpkin Soup

- **Preparation Time:** 45 minutes
- **Serves:** 4

Ingredients:

- 1 small pumpkin peeled, seeded & diced, (about 2 pounds)
- 1 onion, chopped
- 2 cloves garlic, minced
- 2 carrots, peeled and chopped
- 2 stalks celery, chopped
- 4 cups vegetable broth
- 1 teaspoon ground turmeric
- 1/2 teaspoon ground ginger
- 1/2 teaspoon ground cinnamon
- Salt and pepper, to taste

- 1 tablespoon olive oil
- Optional toppings: Greek yogurt, pumpkin seeds, fresh herbs

Nutritional Information: Per serving - Calories: 120kcal | Carbohydrates: 24g | Protein: 3g | Fat: 2g | Saturated Fat: 0g | Cholesterol: 0mg | Sodium: 700mg | Fiber: 5g | Sugar: 9g | Vitamin A: 280% | Vitamin C: 20% | Calcium: 6% | Iron: 8%

Instructions:

1. Preheat the oven to 400°F (200°C).
2. Place the diced pumpkin on a baking sheet lined with parchment paper. Drizzle with olive oil and sprinkle with salt and pepper, toss to coat evenly.
3. Roast the pumpkin in the preheated oven for 25-30 minutes, or until tender and lightly browned.
4. In a large pot, heat olive oil over medium heat, add the chopped onion, garlic, carrots, and celery. Cook for about 5-7 minutes, stirring occasionally, until the vegetables are softened.

5. Add the roasted pumpkin to the pot along with the vegetable broth, ground turmeric, ground ginger, and ground cinnamon. Stir to combine.

6. Bring the soup to a simmer, then reduce the heat to low. Cover and let simmer for 20-25 minutes, allowing the flavors to meld together.

7. Use an immersion blender to blend the soup until smooth. Alternatively, transfer the soup to a blender and blend in batches until smooth, be careful when blending hot liquids.

8. Season the soup with salt and pepper to your preferred taste.

9. Ladle the Detox Roasted Pumpkin Soup into bowls and garnish with optional toppings such as a dollop of Greek yogurt, a sprinkle of pumpkin seeds, and fresh herbs.

10. Serve hot and enjoy the comforting and nutritious flavors of this Detox Roasted Pumpkin Soup!

Serving Suggestions:

- Pair with a slice of whole grain bread or a side salad for a complete and satisfying meal. Enjoy this soup as a delicious and healthy lunch option.

Lemon Parsley Grilled Zucchini

- **Preparation Time:** 15 minutes
- **Serves:** 2

Ingredients:

- 2 medium zucchinis, sliced lengthwise into bout 1/4 inch in thickness
- 2 tablespoons olive oil
- 2 tablespoons freshly squeezed lemon juice
- 2 cloves garlic, minced
- 2 tablespoons chopped fresh parsley
- Salt and pepper, to taste
- Optional garnish: lemon zest

Nutritional Information: Per serving - Calories: 120kcal | Carbohydrates: 7g | Protein: 2g | Fat: 10g | Saturated Fat: 1g | Cholesterol: 0mg | Sodium: 10mg | Fiber: 2g | Sugar:

3g | Vitamin A: 10% | Vitamin C: 40% | Calcium: 4% | Iron: 4%

Instructions:

1. Preheat the grill to medium-high heat.
2. In a small bowl, whisk together the olive oil, lemon juice, minced garlic, chopped fresh parsley, salt, and pepper to make the marinade.
3. Place the sliced zucchini in a shallow dish or large resealable plastic bag. Pour the marinade over the zucchini, ensuring that all the slices are coated evenly. Let marinate for 10-15 minutes.
4. Once the grill is heated, lightly oil the grates to prevent sticking.
5. Place the marinated zucchini slices on the grill in a single layer. Grill for 3-4 minutes on each side, or until tender and grill marks appear.
6. Remove the grilled zucchini from the grill and transfer to a serving platter.
7. Garnish with optional lemon zest before serving, if desired.

8. Serve hot as a delicious and nutritious side dish or as part of a grilled vegetable platter.

Serving Suggestions:

- Pair with grilled chicken, fish, or tofu for a complete and healthy meal. Alternatively, serve it alongside quinoa salad or whole grain couscous for a light and refreshing lunch option.

Spice Rub Grilled Tofu

- **Preparation Time:** 30 minutes (including marinating time)
- **Serves:** 2

Ingredients:

- 1 (14-ounce) piece of extra-firm tofu, squeezed and dried
- 2 tablespoons olive oil

- 1 tablespoon soy sauce or tamari

- 1 tablespoon maple syrup or honey

- 1 teaspoon smoked paprika

- 1/2 teaspoon ground cumin

- 1/2 teaspoon garlic powder

- 1/4 teaspoon chili powder

- Salt and pepper, to taste

- Optional garnish: chopped fresh cilantro or green onions

Nutritional Information: Per serving - Calories: 250kcal | Carbohydrates: 10g | Protein: 16g | Fat: 17g | Saturated Fat: 2g | Cholesterol: 0mg | Sodium: 360mg | Fiber: 1g | Sugar: 6g | Vitamin A: 4% | Vitamin C: 0% | Calcium: 25% | Iron: 15%

Instructions:

1. Preheat the grill to medium-high heat.

2. In a small bowl, whisk together the olive oil, soy sauce or tamari, maple syrup or honey, smoked paprika, ground cumin, garlic powder, chili powder, salt, and pepper to make the spice rub marinade.

3. Slice the pressed and drained tofu block into 1/2-inch thick slices.

4. Place the tofu slices in a shallow dish or large resealable plastic bag, pour the spice rub marinade over the tofu, ensuring that all slices are coated evenly.

5. Let marinate for at least 15-20 minutes, once the grill is heated, lightly oil the grates to prevent sticking.

6. Carefully place the marinated tofu slices on the grill. Grill for 3-4 minutes on each side, or until grill marks appear and the tofu is heated through.

7. Remove the grilled tofu from the grill and transfer to a serving platter.

8. Garnish with chopped fresh cilantro or green onions before serving, if desired.

9. Serve hot as a protein-rich main dish or as a delicious addition to salads, bowls, or sandwiches.

Serving Suggestions:

- Pair this Spice Rub Grilled Tofu with grilled vegetables, brown rice, or quinoa for a balanced and nutritious meal.

  Alternatively, use the grilled tofu slices as a filling for tacos or wraps, or chop them up and toss them into stir-fries or noodle dishes.

Dinner Recipes for Fatty Liver Diet

Herb-Infused Quinoa Medley

- **Preparation Time:** 25 minutes
- **Serves:** 4

Ingredients:

- 1 cup quinoa, rinsed
- 2 cups vegetable broth
- 1 tablespoon olive oil
- 1 onion, finely chopped
- 2 cloves garlic, minced
- 1 bell pepper, diced

- 1 zucchini, diced

- 1 carrot, diced

- 1 teaspoon dried thyme

- 1 teaspoon dried oregano

- Salt and pepper, to taste

- 1/4 cup chopped fresh parsley

- Lemon wedges, for serving

Nutritional Information: Per serving - Calories: 240kcal | Carbohydrates: 40g | Protein: 7g | Fat: 6g | Saturated Fat: 1g | Cholesterol: 0mg | Sodium: 580mg | Fiber: 6g | Sugar: 5g | Vitamin A: 90% | Vitamin C: 70% | Calcium: 6% | Iron: 15%

Instructions:

1. In a fine mesh strainer, rinse the quinoa under cold water until the water runs clear. This will remove any bitterness from the quinoa.

2. In a medium saucepan, bring the vegetable broth to a boil, add the rinsed quinoa, reduce the heat to low, cover, and simmer for 15-20 minutes, or until the quinoa is fluffy and the liquid is absorbed.

3. Remove from heat, let it sit and covered, for 5 minutes.

4. In a large skillet, heat olive oil over medium heat, add chopped onion and minced garlic, and sauté until softened and fragrant, about 3-4 minutes.

5. Add diced bell pepper, zucchini, and carrot to the skillet, and cook until the vegetables are tender yet still slightly crisp, about 5-6 minutes.

6. Stir in dried thyme, dried oregano, salt, and pepper, and cook for another 1-2 minutes, allowing the herbs to become fragrant.

7. Fluff the cooked quinoa with a fork and add it to the skillet with the vegetable mixture, stir well to combine and heat through.

8. Remove the skillet from heat and stir in chopped fresh parsley.

9. Transfer the Herb-Infused Quinoa Medley to a serving dish and garnish with lemon wedges.

10. Serve hot as a flavorful and nutritious side dish or light vegetarian main course.

Serving Suggestions:

- Serve alongside grilled tofu or roasted chickpeas for added protein and texture. Pair it with a mixed green salad dressed with lemon tahini dressing for a refreshing and balanced meal.

Turkey Burger Bowl Salad

- **Preparation Time:** 20 minutes
- **Serves**: 2

Ingredients:

- 1 lb. ground turkey
- 1 tablespoon olive oil
- 1 teaspoon garlic powder
- 1 teaspoon onion powder
- Salt and pepper to taste
- 4 cups mixed salad greens
- 1 cup cherry tomatoes, halved
- 1 cucumber, sliced
- 1/2 red onion, thinly sliced

- 1 avocado, diced
- 1/4 cup crumbled feta cheese
- Balsamic vinaigrette dressing, for serving

Nutritional Information: Per serving - Calories: 450kcal, Carbohydrates: 18g, Protein: 30g, Fat: 30g, Fiber: 8g, Sugar: 7g, Vitamin A: 120%, Vitamin C: 70%, Calcium: 15%, Iron: 20%

Instructions:

1. In a mixing bowl, combine the ground turkey with garlic powder, onion powder, salt, and pepper, form the mixture into two burger patties.
2. Heat olive oil in a skillet over medium heat, cook the turkey burgers for 4-5 minutes on each side, or until they are cooked through and reach an internal temperature of 165°F.
3. While the burgers are cooking, prepare the salad ingredients, divide the mixed salad greens between two serving bowls.
4. Top the salad greens with cherry tomatoes, cucumber slices, red onion slices, diced avocado, and crumbled feta cheese.

5. Once the turkey burgers are cooked, place them on top of the salad bowls.

6. Drizzle balsamic vinaigrette dressing over the salad bowls.

7. Serve the Turkey Burger Bowl Salads immediately, and enjoy.

Serving Suggestions:

- For an extra burst of flavor, sprinkle some freshly chopped herbs like parsley or basil over the salad before serving. You can also add additional toppings such as roasted nuts or seeds for added crunch.

Eggplant & Lentil Bake

- **Preparation Time:** 1 hour
- **Serves:** 4

Ingredients:

- 1 large eggplant, sliced into rounds

- 1 cup dry green lentils (thoroughly rinsed & drained)
- 2 cups vegetable broth
- 1 onion, chopped
- 2 cloves garlic, minced
- 14 oz. (1 can) diced tomatoes, drained
- 1 teaspoon dried oregano
- 1 teaspoon dried basil
- Salt and pepper, to taste
- 1 cup shredded mozzarella cheese
- Fresh basil leaves, for garnish

Nutritional Information: Per serving - Calories: 280kcal | Carbohydrates: 38g | Protein: 17g | Fat: 7g | Saturated Fat: 3g | Cholesterol: 15mg | Sodium: 700mg | Fiber: 15g | Sugar: 8g | Vitamin A: 15% | Vitamin C: 20% | Calcium: 20% | Iron: 25%

Instructions:

1. Preheat your oven to 375°F (190°C).
2. Place the sliced eggplant rounds on a baking sheet lined with parchment paper.

3. Sprinkle both sides of the eggplant slices with salt and let them sit for about 15 minutes to draw out excess moisture, pat the eggplant slices dry with paper towels, after 15 minutes.

4. In a medium saucepan, combine the rinsed lentils and vegetable broth. Bring to a boil, then reduce the heat to low, cover, and simmer for about 20-25 minutes, or until the lentils are tender and the liquid is absorbed.

5. In a skillet, heat a tablespoon of olive oil over medium heat, add the chopped onion and cook until softened, about 5 minutes. Add the minced garlic and cook for extra minutes.

6. Add the drained diced tomatoes, dried oregano, and dried basil to the skillet.

7. Season with salt and pepper to taste, cook for about 5 minutes, allowing the flavors to meld together.

8. In a greased baking dish, layer half of the cooked lentils followed by half of the tomato mixture.

9. Then, arrange half of the eggplant slices on top, repeat the layers with the remaining lentils, tomato mixture, and eggplant slices.

10. Sprinkle the shredded mozzarella cheese evenly over the top of the casserole, cover the baking dish with aluminum foil and bake in the preheated oven for 25-30 minutes, or until the cheese is melted and bubbly.

11. Remove the foil and bake for an additional 5-10 minutes, or until the cheese is golden brown.

12. Garnish with fresh basil leaves before serving.

Serving Suggestions:

- Serve as a main dish alongside a green salad dressed with balsamic vinaigrette for a complete meal.

  Pair it with garlic bread or whole grain rolls for a satisfying dinner option.

Green Goddess Supper

- **Preparation Time:** 30 minutes
- **Serves:** 4

Ingredients:

- 8 ounces' whole wheat spaghetti

- 2 cups broccoli florets

- 1 cup green peas

- 1 tablespoon olive oil

- 2 cloves garlic, minced

- 1 cup spinach leaves

- 1 avocado, diced

- 1/4 cup fresh basil leaves

- 1/4 cup fresh parsley leaves

- Juice of 1 lemon

- Salt and pepper, to taste

- Grated Parmesan cheese, for serving (optional)

Nutritional Information: Per serving - Calories: 350kcal | Carbohydrates: 55g | Protein: 13g | Fat: 11g | Saturated Fat: 2g | Cholesterol: 0mg | Sodium: 80mg | Fiber: 11g | Sugar: 4g | Vitamin A: 40% | Vitamin C: 90% | Calcium: 10% | Iron: 20%

Instructions:

1. Cook the whole wheat spaghetti according to the package instructions until al dente. During the last 3 minutes of cooking, add the broccoli florets and

green peas to the boiling water. Drain the pasta and vegetables, reserving 1/2 cup of the cooking water.

2. In a large skillet, heat olive oil over medium heat, add minced garlic and sauté for 1-2 minutes until fragrant.

3. Add the cooked spaghetti, broccoli, and peas to the skillet, along with the reserved cooking water. Stir in spinach leaves and cook for 2-3 minutes until the spinach is wilted.

4. In a blender or food processor, combine diced avocado, basil leaves, parsley leaves, lemon juice, salt, and pepper. Blend until smooth and creamy.

5. Pour the avocado sauce over the pasta and vegetables in the skillet. Toss gently to coat everything evenly.

6. Remove the skillet from heat and serve the Green Goddess Supper immediately.

7. Garnish with grated Parmesan cheese, if desired.

Serving Suggestions:

- Enjoy the Green Goddess Supper as a nutritious and satisfying meal on its own, or serve it alongside a simple green salad dressed with lemon vinaigrette

Barley-Stuffed Poblanos/Peppers

- **Preparation Time:** 1 hour
- **Serves:** 4

Ingredients:

- 4 large poblano peppers
- 1 cup pearl barley
- 2 cups vegetable broth
- 1 tablespoon olive oil
- 1 onion, diced
- 2 cloves garlic, minced
- 1 carrot, diced
- 1 zucchini, diced
- 14 oz. black beans (drained & rinsed)
- 1 cup corn kernels (fresh, frozen, or canned)
- 1 teaspoon ground cumin
- 1 teaspoon chili powder
- Salt and pepper, to taste

- 1/2 cup shredded cheddar cheese (optional)
- Fresh cilantro, chopped, for garnish

Nutritional Information: Per serving - Calories: 380kcal | Carbohydrates: 68g | Protein: 15g | Fat: 7g | Saturated Fat: 2g | Cholesterol: 5mg | Sodium: 800mg | Fiber: 14g | Sugar: 7g | Vitamin A: 120% | Vitamin C: 150% | Calcium: 15% | Iron: 25%

Instructions:

1. Preheat your oven to 400°F (200°C), line a baking sheet with parchment paper.
2. Cut the tops off the poblano peppers and remove the seeds and membranes. Place the peppers on the prepared baking sheet and set aside.
3. In a medium saucepan, bring the vegetable broth to a boil, add the pearl barley, reduce the heat to low, cover, and simmer for 30-35 minutes, or until the barley is done and the liquid is absorbed.
4. Heat the olive oil over medium heat in a large skillet, add the diced onion and cook until softened, about 5 minutes.

5. Add the minced garlic, diced carrot, and diced zucchini to the skillet, cook for another 5 minutes, or until the vegetables are tender.

6. Stir in the cooked pearl barley, black beans, corn kernels, ground cumin, and chili powder. Season with salt and pepper to taste, cook for extra 5 minutes, allowing the flavors to meld together.

7. Spoon the barley and vegetable mixture into the prepared poblano peppers, dividing it evenly among them.

8. If desired, sprinkle shredded cheddar cheese over the stuffed peppers.

9. Bake in the preheated oven for 20-25 minutes, or until the peppers are tender and the filling is heated through.

10. Remove from the oven and garnish with chopped fresh cilantro before serving.

Serving Suggestions:

- Pair with a side salad dressed with lime vinaigrette for a refreshing contrast to the spicy peppers.

Spaghetti Squash Bolognese

- **Preparation Time:** 1 hour
- **Serves:** 4

Ingredients:

- 1 medium spaghetti squash
- 1 tablespoon olive oil
- 1 onion, diced
- 2 cloves garlic, minced
- 1 carrot, diced
- 1 celery stalk, diced
- 8 oz. lean ground turkey or beef
- 1 can (14 oz.) diced tomatoes
- 1 tablespoon tomato paste
- 1 teaspoon dried oregano
- 1 teaspoon dried basil
- Salt and pepper, to taste
- Fresh parsley, chopped, for garnish
- Grated Parmesan cheese, for serving (optional)

Nutritional Information: Per serving - Calories: 230kcal | Carbohydrates: 24g | Protein: 15g | Fat: 10g | Saturated Fat: 3g | Cholesterol: 35mg | Sodium: 460mg | Fiber: 6g

Instructions:

1. Preheat your oven to 400°F (200°C), line a baking sheet with parchment paper.

2. Cut the spaghetti squash in half lengthwise and scoop out the seeds with a spoon, drizzle the cut sides with olive oil and season with salt and pepper.

3. Arrange the squash on the prepared baking sheet with the cut sides down.

4. Bake in the preheated oven for 35-45 minutes, or until the squash is tender and easily pierced with a fork, remove from the oven and let it cool slightly.

5. While the squash is baking, heat the olive oil in a large skillet over medium heat, add the diced onion, minced garlic, diced carrot, and diced celery. Cook until the vegetables are softened, about 5-6 minutes.

6. Add the lean ground beef or turkey to the skillet. Cook, breaking it apart with a spoon, until it is cooked through and browned.

7. Stir in the diced tomatoes, tomato paste, dried oregano, dried basil, salt, and pepper. Simmer for 15-20 minutes, until the sauce has thickened and the flavors have combined.

8. Using a fork, scrape the cooked spaghetti squash strands from the shells into a large bowl.

9. Serve the spaghetti squash topped with the Bolognese sauce, garnish with chopped fresh parsley and grated Parmesan cheese, if desired.

Serving Suggestions:

- Serve this Spaghetti Squash Bolognese hot as a lighter and healthier alternative to traditional pasta dishes.

  Enjoy the savory and flavorful Bolognese sauce paired with the tender strands of spaghetti squash.

Lebanese Kafta Kebabs with Tahini Sauce

- **Preparation Time:** 45 minutes
- **Serves:** 4

Ingredients:

For the Kafta Kebabs:

- 1 lb. ground lamb or beef
- 1 onion, finely chopped
- 2 cloves garlic, minced
- 1/4 cup fresh parsley, finely chopped
- 1/4 cup fresh mint, finely chopped
- 1 teaspoon ground cumin
- 1 teaspoon ground coriander
- 1/2 teaspoon paprika
- Salt and pepper, to taste
- Wooden skewers, soaked in water for 30 minutes

For the Tahini Sauce:

- 1/2 cup tahini paste
- 1/4 cup water
- 2 tablespoons lemon juice
- 1 clove garlic, minced
- Salt, to taste

Optional Garnish:

- Chopped fresh parsley or mint
- Sumac

Nutritional Information: Per serving (including tahini sauce) - Calories: 420kcal | Carbohydrates: 10g | Protein: 23g | Fat: 33g | Saturated Fat: 8g | Cholesterol: 70mg | Sodium: 90mg | Fiber: 3g | Sugar: 1g | Vitamin A: 10% | Vitamin C: 15% | Calcium: 10% | Iron: 20%

Instructions:

1. In a large mixing bowl, combine the ground lamb or beef, finely chopped onion, minced garlic, chopped parsley, chopped mint, ground cumin, ground coriander, paprika, salt, and pepper. Mix until well combined.

2. Divide the meat mixture into equal portions and shape each portion onto a wooden skewer, forming elongated sausage-like shapes. Press the meat firmly around the skewers to prevent them from falling off during grilling.

3. Set your grill or grill pan to a moderately high temperature.

4. Place the kafta kebabs on the preheated grill and cook for 4-5 minutes on each side, or until they are browned and cooked through.

5. While the kebabs are cooking, prepare the tahini sauce. In a small bowl, whisk together the tahini paste, water, lemon juice, minced garlic, and salt until smooth and creamy.

6. If the sauce is too thick, add more water until desired consistency is reached, once the kafta kebabs are cooked, remove them from the grill and let them rest for a few minutes.

7. Serve the kafta kebabs hot with the tahini sauce drizzled over the top.

8. Garnish with chopped fresh parsley or mint and a sprinkle of sumac, if desired.

Serving Suggestions:

- Serve these Lebanese Kafta Kebabs with Tahini Sauce hot off the grill as a main dish, accompanied by warm pita bread, hummus, tabbouleh, and a side salad for a complete and satisfying meal.

Desserts and Snacks for Fatty Liver Diet

Baked Bhakarwadi

- **Preparation Time:** 1 hour 30 minutes
- **Serves:** 6

Ingredients:

For the dough:

- 1 cup chickpea flour (besan)
- 1 cup all-purpose flour
- 2 tablespoons semolina (sooji)
- 2 tablespoons oil
- Water, as needed

For the filling:

- 1 cup grated coconut
- 1/2 cup roasted sesame seeds
- 1/4 cup chopped peanuts
- 2 tablespoons poppy seeds (khus khus)
- 1 tablespoon ginger paste

- 1 tablespoon garlic paste

- 1 tablespoon green chili paste

- 1 teaspoon turmeric powder

- 1 teaspoon garam masala

- 1 teaspoon ground coriander

- Salt, to taste

- 2 tablespoons oil

For brushing:

- 2 tablespoons melted ghee or oil

Nutritional Information: Per serving - Calories: 320kcal | Carbohydrates: 30g | Protein: 8g | Fat: 20g | Saturated Fat: 8g | Cholesterol: 0mg | Sodium: 150mg | Fiber: 6g | Sugar: 2g | Vitamin A: 0% | Vitamin C: 2% | Calcium: 8% | Iron: 15%

Instructions:

1. In a mixing bowl, combine chickpea flour, all-purpose flour, semolina, and oil. Gradually add

water and knead into a smooth dough, cover and let it rest for 30 minutes.

2. Meanwhile, prepare the filling. In a pan, heat oil and add grated coconut, roasted sesame seeds, chopped peanuts, poppy seeds, ginger paste, garlic paste, green chili paste, turmeric powder, garam masala, ground coriander, and salt.

3. Cook until the mixture is aromatic and slightly browned, remove from heat and let it cool.

4. Preheat the oven to 350°F (180°C), line a baking sheet with parchment paper.

5. Divide the dough into small portions and roll each portion into a thin circle.

6. Spread a layer of the prepared filling onto each dough circle and roll it tightly to form a log.

7. Slice the rolled dough into 1-inch pieces.

8. Place the slices on the prepared baking sheet and brush them with melted ghee or oil.

9. Bake in the preheated oven for 20-25 minutes, or until golden brown and crispy.

10. Take them out of the oven and let them cool slightly before serving.

Serving Suggestions:

- Serve the Baked Bhakarwadi as a crunchy and flavorful snack alongside a hot cup of masala chai or a tangy tamarind chutney.

Celery Sticks with Hummus

- **Preparation Time:** 10 minutes
- **Serves:** 4

Ingredients:

- 4 celery stalks, trimmed and cut into sticks
- 1 cup hummus (store-bought or homemade)

Nutritional Information: Per serving - Calories: 150kcal | Carbohydrates: 10g | Protein: 6g | Fat: 10g | Saturated Fat: 1g | Cholesterol: 0mg | Sodium: 300mg | Fiber: 5g | Sugar: 2g | Vitamin A: 10% | Vitamin C: 6% | Calcium: 4% | Iron: 10%

Instructions:

1. Wash and trim the celery stalks, then cut them into sticks of desired size.

2. Place the celery sticks on a serving platter.

3. Serve the celery sticks with hummus on the side for dipping.

Serving Suggestions:

- Enjoy the Celery Sticks with Hummus as a healthy and crunchy snack option. Pair it with other sliced vegetables like carrots, bell peppers, and cucumber for a colorful and nutritious snack platter.

Chocolate Fudge Pie

- **Preparation Time:** 30 minutes
- **Serves:** 8

Ingredients:

- 1 9-inch pie crust (either homemade or purchased from a store)
- 1 cup dark chocolate chips
- 1/2 cup unsweetened cocoa powder
- 1/2 cup maple syrup or honey
- 1/4 cup coconut oil, melted
- 1 teaspoon vanilla extract

- Pinch of salt

- Optional toppings: sliced strawberries, raspberries, or whipped coconut cream

Nutritional Information: Per serving - Calories: 320kcal | Carbohydrates: 30g | Protein: 4g | Fat: 22g | Saturated Fat: 15g | Cholesterol: 0mg | Sodium: 120mg | Fiber: 5g | Sugar: 18g | Vitamin A: 0% | Vitamin C: 0% | Calcium: 4% | Iron: 15%

Instructions:

1. Preheat your oven to 350°F (175°C). Place the pie crust in a 9-inch pie dish and crimp the edges, use a fork to prick holes in the bottom of the crust.

2. Bake the pie crust in the preheated oven for 10-12 minutes, or until lightly golden brown, remove from the oven and let it cool completely.

3. In a microwave-safe bowl, combine the dark chocolate chips, unsweetened cocoa powder, maple syrup or honey, melted coconut oil, vanilla extract, and a pinch of salt.

4. Microwave the mixture in 30-second intervals, stirring after each interval, until the chocolate chips are melted and the mixture is smooth.

5. Pour the chocolate fudge mixture into the cooled pie crust and spread it out evenly.

6. Refrigerate the pie for at least 2 hours, or until the filling is set.

7. Once set, remove the pie from the refrigerator and let it sit at room temperature for 5-10 minutes before slicing.

8. Slice the chocolate fudge pie into wedges and serve with optional toppings like sliced strawberries, raspberries, or whipped coconut cream.

Serving Suggestions:

- Indulge in this decadent Chocolate Fudge Pie as a rich and satisfying dessert option.
  Serve it at room temperature or slightly chilled, and top it with fresh berries or a dollop of whipped coconut cream for an extra special touch.

Tzatziki Dip with Baby Carrots

- **Preparation Time:** 15 minutes
- **Serves:** 4

Ingredients:

- 1 cup Greek yogurt
- 1 cucumber, grated and squeezed to remove excess moisture
- 2 cloves garlic, minced
- 1 tablespoon fresh lemon juice
- 1 tablespoon extra-virgin olive oil
- 1 tablespoon chopped fresh dill
- Salt and pepper, to taste
- Baby carrots, for dipping

Nutritional Information: Per serving (dip only) - Calories: 70kcal | Carbohydrates: 4g | Protein: 4g | Fat: 4g | Saturated Fat: 1g | Cholesterol: 5mg | Sodium: 30mg | Fiber: 1g | Sugar: 3g | Vitamin A: 8% | Vitamin C: 6% | Calcium: 6% | Iron: 2%

Instructions:

1. In a mixing bowl, combine Greek yogurt, grated cucumber, minced garlic, fresh lemon juice, extra virgin olive oil, chopped fresh dill, salt, and pepper. Stir until well combined.

2. Taste and adjust seasoning, if needed, by adding more salt, pepper, or lemon juice to taste.

3. Transfer the tzatziki dip to a serving bowl.

4. Arrange baby carrots on a serving platter around the bowl of tzatziki dip.

Serving Suggestions:

- Serve the Tzatziki Dip with Baby Carrots as a refreshing and healthy snack option. The creamy and tangy tzatziki pairs perfectly with the crisp and sweet baby carrots, making it a delicious and nutritious dip for any occasion.

Peanut Butter Cookies

- **Preparation Time:** 20 minutes
- **Serves:** 12 cookies

Ingredients:

- 1 cup natural peanut butter (smooth or with bits)
- 1/2 cup coconut sugar or brown sugar
- 1 large egg
- 1 teaspoon vanilla extract
- 1/2 teaspoon baking soda
- Pinch of salt

Nutritional Information: Per serving (1 cookie) - Calories: 150kcal | Carbohydrates: 9g | Protein: 6g | Fat: 11g | Saturated Fat: 2g | Cholesterol: 15mg | Sodium: 100mg | Fiber: 1g | Sugar: 6g | Vitamin A: 0% | Vitamin C: 0% | Calcium: 0% | Iron: 2%

Instructions:

1. Set your oven to 350°F (175°C), cover a baking sheet with parchment paper.

2. In a mixing bowl, combine the natural peanut butter, coconut sugar or brown sugar, egg, vanilla extract, baking soda, and a pinch of salt. Mix until it is well combined.

3. Scoop out tablespoon-sized portions of the cookie dough and roll them into balls. Place the balls on the prepared baking sheet, leaving space between each cookie.

4. Use a fork to flatten each cookie slightly and create a crisscross pattern on top.

5. Bake the cookies in the preheated oven for 8-10 minutes, or until lightly golden brown around the edges.

6. Remove the cookies from the oven and let them cool on the baking sheet for a while before moving them to a cooling rack to cool completely.

Serving Suggestions:

- Serve them alongside a glass of almond milk or a cup of your favorite herbal tea for a comforting treat.

Beverages/Drinks for Fatty Liver Diet

Mango Mint Iced Green Tea

- **Preparation Time:** 15 minutes
- **Serves:** 4

Ingredients:

- 4 cups water
- 4 green tea bags
- 1 ripe mango, peeled and diced
- 1/4 cup fresh mint leaves
- 2 tablespoons honey or maple syrup (if desired)
- Ice cubes
- For garnish: Mint sprigs & mango slices

Nutritional Information: Per serving - Calories: 30kcal | Carbohydrates: 8g | Fiber: 1g | Sugars: 6g | Vitamin C: 25% | Calcium: 2% | Iron: 2%

Instructions:

1. Boil water in a medium saucepan, remove the saucepan from heat and add the green tea bags.

2. Let the tea steep for about 3-5 minutes, depending on your desired strength.

3. Meanwhile, in a blender, combine the diced mango, fresh mint leaves, and honey or maple syrup (if using). Blend until smooth.

4. Once the green tea has steeped, remove the tea bags and discard them.

5. Pour the mango-mint puree into the saucepan with the green tea. Stir well to combine.

6. Allow the mixture to cool to room temperature, then transfer it to the refrigerator to chill for at least 1 hour.

7. To serve, fill glasses with ice cubes and pour the chilled mango-mint green tea over the ice.

8. Garnish each glass with a mint sprig and a slice of mango.

9. Serve immediately and enjoy the refreshing Mango Mint Iced Green Tea!

Serving Suggestions:

- You can add a splash of sparkling water for an extra fizzy twist.

Pomegranate Juice

- **Preparation Time:** 10 minutes
- **Serves:** 2

Ingredients:

- 2 large pomegranates
- Water (optional, for diluting)
- Ice cubes
- Fresh mint leaves, for garnish (optional)

Nutritional Information: Per serving (without added water) - Calories: 140kcal | Carbohydrates: 33g | Fiber: 7g | Sugars: 24g | Vitamin C: 48% | Vitamin K: 46% | Potassium: 12%

Instructions:

1. Cut the pomegranates in half and extract the seeds (arils) by gently tapping the back of each half with a wooden spoon over a bowl. Collect all the seeds in the bowl.
2. Transfer the pomegranate seeds to a blender or food processor.

3. Blend the pomegranate seeds on high speed until smooth.

4. Place a fine mesh strainer over a bowl or pitcher. Pour the blended pomegranate mixture through the strainer to remove the pulp and extract the juice.

5. Use the back of a spoon to press down on the pulp in the strainer, extracting as much juice as possible.

6. Discard the remaining pulp and transfer the strained pomegranate juice to serving glasses filled with ice cubes.

7. Optionally, you can dilute the pomegranate juice with water to your desired taste and consistency.

8. Garnish the glasses with fresh mint leaves, if desired.

9. Serve the refreshing Pomegranate Juice immediately and enjoy!

Serving Suggestions:

- Enjoy the Pomegranate Juice as a nutritious and antioxidant-rich beverage on its own, or use it as a base for cocktails and mocktails.

Beetroot Juice

- **Preparation Time:** 10 minutes
- **Serves:** 2

Ingredients:

- 2 medium-sized beetroots, peeled and chopped
- 1 large apple, cored and chopped
- 1 medium-sized carrot, peeled and chopped
- 1-inch piece of ginger, peeled
- 1 lemon, juiced
- Water (optional, for diluting)
- Ice cubes

Nutritional Information: Per serving (without added water) - Calories: 110kcal | Carbohydrates: 27g | Fiber: 6g | Sugars: 17g | Vitamin A: 130% | Vitamin C: 60% | Iron: 6% | Calcium: 4%

Instructions:

1. Place the chopped beetroots, apple, carrot, and ginger into a juicer.

2. Juice all the ingredients according to the juicer's instructions until smooth.

3. Once juiced, add the lemon juice to the mixture and stir well to combine.

4. If the juice is too thick, you can dilute it with water to your desired consistency.

5. Pour the Beetroot Juice into serving glasses filled with ice cubes.

6. Optionally, you can garnish with a slice of lemon or a sprig of mint.

7. Serve the refreshing Beetroot Juice immediately and enjoy.

Serving Suggestions:

- Beetroot Juice is a vibrant and nutritious beverage that can be enjoyed on its own or as part of a juice cleanse. This refreshing juice is perfect for promoting overall health and well-being.

Pu-erh Tea

- **Preparation Time:** 5 minutes
- **Serves:** 1

Ingredients:

- Pu-erh tea leaves (compressed or loose)
- Water

Nutritional Information: Per serving - Calories: 0 | Carbohydrates: 0g | Protein: 0g | Fat: 0g | Fiber: 0g | Sugar: 0g

Instructions:

1. Boil water in a kettle or pot, the ideal temperature for Pu-erh tea is around 195-205°F (90-96°C).
2. Rinse your teapot or teacup with hot water to warm it up.
3. If you're using compressed Pu-erh tea, break off a small piece (about 5-10 grams) from the tea cake or brick. If you're using loose Pu-erh tea, measure out the desired amount (about 1-2 teaspoons per cup).

4. Place the Pu-erh tea leaves into the warmed teapot or teacup.

5. Pour the hot water over the tea leaves, covering them completely.

6. Allow the Pu-erh tea to steep for 3-5 minutes, depending on your preference for strength.

7. Once steeped, strain the tea leaves or remove the infuser from the teapot.

8. Pour the brewed Pu-erh tea into a serving cup.

9. Enjoy the rich and earthy flavor of Pu-erh tea on its own or with a slice of lemon or a splash of milk, if desired.

Serving Suggestions:

- Pu-erh tea can be enjoyed as a standalone beverage, sipped slowly to appreciate its unique flavor profile. Experiment with different brewing methods and steeping times to find your preferred way of enjoying Pu-erh tea.

Peach Smoothies

- **Preparation Time:** 5 minutes
- **Serves:** 2

Ingredients:

- 2 ripe peaches, pitted and chopped
- 1 banana, peeled and sliced
- 1/2 cup Greek yogurt
- 1/2 cup almond milk (or any milk you want)
- 1 tablespoon honey or maple syrup (if desired)
- Ice cubes

Nutritional Information: Per serving - Calories: 150kcal | Carbohydrates: 34g | Protein: 5g | Fat: 1g | Fiber: 4g | Sugar: 26g | Vitamin C: 15% | Calcium: 10% | Iron: 2%

Instructions:

1. Place the chopped peaches, sliced banana, Greek yogurt, almond milk, and honey or maple syrup (if using) into a blender.
2. Add a handful of ice cubes to the blender to make the smoothie cold and refreshing.

3. Blend all the ingredients until smooth and creamy, scraping down the sides of the blender as needed.

4. Once the smoothie reaches your desired consistency, taste and adjust the sweetness if necessary by adding more honey or maple syrup.

5. Pour the Peach Smoothies into serving glasses.

6. Optionally, garnish each glass with a slice of peach or a sprinkle of cinnamon for extra flavor.

7. Serve the refreshing Peach Smoothies immediately and enjoy!

Serving Suggestions:

- You can customize the smoothie by adding a handful of spinach or kale for added greens, or a scoop of protein powder for an extra protein boost.

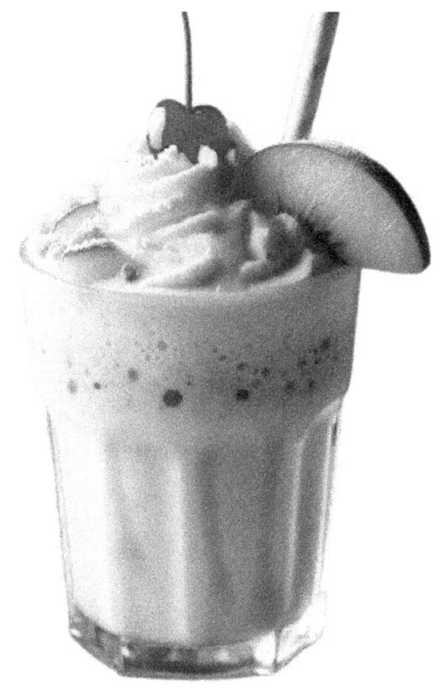

CHAPTER 3

30 Days Meal Plan for Fatty Liver Diet

Please note that the provided meal plan is a sample and should not be interpreted as a recommendation to consume all the listed recipes in a single day.

This meal plan aims to offer inspiration and guidance for healthy meal preparation. Feel free to customize this plan to suit your preferences and dietary requirements.

Day 1:

- **Breakfast:** Chia seeds pudding with berries and coconut flakes
- **Lunch:** Chicken and Vegetable Wrap with Ginger Sauce
- **Dinner:** Herb-Infused Quinoa Medley
- **Dessert/Snack:** Baked Bhakarwadi
- **Beverage:** Mango Mint Iced Green Tea

Day 2:

- **Breakfast:** Viking Crispbread with salmon
- **Lunch:** Tuna Salad Stuffed Tomato with Whole Grain Crackers
- **Dinner:** Eggplant & Lentil Bake
- **Dessert/Snack:** Celery sticks with hummus
- **Beverage:** Pomegranate Juice

Day 3:

- **Breakfast:** Walnut or Pecan Apple Oatmeal
- **Lunch:** Sweet Potato and Black Bean Tacos
- **Dinner:** Turkey Burger Bowl Salad
- **Dessert/Snack:** Chocolate Fudge Pie
- **Beverage:** Peach Smoothie

Day 4:

- **Breakfast:** Blueberry and Granola Yogurt Parfait
- **Lunch:** Mushroom and Spinach Quesadillas
- **Dinner:** Green Goddess Supper
- **Dessert/Snack:** Tzatziki dip with baby carrot
- **Beverage:** Beetroot Juice

Day 5:

- **Breakfast:** Toast with avocados and ricotta
- **Lunch:** Detox Roasted Pumpkin Soup
- **Dinner:** Barley-Stuffed Poblanos/Peppers
- **Dessert/Snack:** Peanut Butter Cookies
- **Beverage:** Pu-erh tea

Day 6:

- **Breakfast:** Cheese and Veggie Egg White Breakfast Sandwich
- **Lunch:** Lemon Parsley Grilled Zucchini
- **Dinner:** Spaghetti Squash Bolognese
- **Dessert/Snack:** Baked Bhakarwadi
- **Beverage:** Mango Mint Iced Green Tea

Day 7:

- **Breakfast:** Cheerios and Almond Milk Bowl
- **Lunch:** Spice Rub Grilled Tofu
- **Dinner:** Lebanese Kafta Kebabs with Tahini Sauce
- **Dessert/Snack:** Celery sticks with hummus
- **Beverage:** Pomegranate Juice

Day 8:

- **Breakfast:** Chia seeds pudding with berries and coconut flakes
- **Lunch:** Chicken and Vegetable Wrap with Ginger Sauce
- **Dinner:** Herb-Infused Quinoa Medley
- **Dessert/Snack:** Chocolate Fudge Pie
- **Beverage:** Beetroot Juice

Day 9:

- **Breakfast:** Viking Crispbread with salmon
- **Lunch:** Tuna Salad Stuffed Tomato with Whole Grain Crackers
- **Dinner:** Eggplant & Lentil Bake
- **Dessert/Snack:** Peanut Butter Cookies
- **Beverage:** Pu-erh tea

Day 10:

- **Breakfast:** Walnut or Pecan Apple Oatmeal
- **Lunch:** Sweet Potato and Black Bean Tacos
- **Dinner:** Turkey Burger Bowl Salad

- **Dessert/Snack:** Baked Bhakarwadi

- **Beverage:** Mango Mint Iced Green Tea

Day 11:

- **Breakfast:** Blueberry and Granola Yogurt Parfait

- **Lunch:** Mushroom and Spinach Quesadillas

- **Dinner:** Green Goddess Supper

- **Dessert/Snack:** Tzatziki dip with baby carrot

- **Beverage:** Pomegranate Juice

Day 12:

- **Breakfast:** Toast with avocados and ricotta

- **Lunch:** Detox Roasted Pumpkin Soup

- **Dinner:** Barley-Stuffed Poblanos/Peppers

- **Dessert/Snack:** Celery sticks with hummus

- **Beverage:** Peach Smoothie

Day 13:

- **Breakfast:** Cheese and Veggie Egg White Breakfast Sandwich

- **Lunch:** Lemon Parsley Grilled Zucchini

- **Dinner:** Spaghetti Squash Bolognese

- **Dessert/Snack:** Chocolate Fudge Pie

- **Beverage:** Beetroot Juice

Day 14:

- **Breakfast:** Cheerios and Almond Milk Bowl

- **Lunch:** Spice Rub Grilled Tofu

- **Dinner:** Lebanese Kafta Kebabs with Tahini Sauce

- **Dessert/Snack:** Peanut Butter Cookies

- **Beverage:** Pu-erh tea

Day 15:

- **Breakfast:** Chia seeds pudding with berries and coconut flakes

- **Lunch:** Chicken and Vegetable Wrap with Ginger Sauce

- **Dinner:** Herb-Infused Quinoa Medley

- **Dessert/Snack:** Tzatziki dip with baby carrot

- **Beverage:** Mango Mint Iced Green Tea

Day 16:

- **Breakfast:** Viking Crispbread with salmon

- **Lunch:** Tuna Salad Stuffed Tomato with Whole Grain Crackers
- **Dinner:** Eggplant & Lentil Bake
- **Dessert/Snack:** Baked Bhakarwadi
- **Beverage:** Pomegranate Juice

Day 17:

- **Breakfast:** Walnut or Pecan Apple Oatmeal
- **Lunch:** Sweet Potato and Black Bean Tacos
- **Dinner:** Turkey Burger Bowl Salad
- **Dessert/Snack:** Celery sticks with hummus
- **Beverage:** Peach Smoothie

Day 18:

- **Breakfast:** Blueberry and Granola Yogurt Parfait
- **Lunch:** Mushroom and Spinach Quesadillas
- **Dinner:** Green Goddess Supper
- **Dessert/Snack:** Chocolate Fudge Pie
- **Beverage:** Beetroot Juice

Day 19:

- **Breakfast:** Toast with avocados and ricotta
- **Lunch:** Detox Roasted Pumpkin Soup
- **Dinner:** Barley-Stuffed Poblanos/Peppers
- **Dessert/Snack:** Peanut Butter Cookies
- **Beverage:** Pu-erh tea

Day 20:

- **Breakfast:** Cheese and Veggie Egg White Breakfast Sandwich
- **Lunch:** Lemon Parsley Grilled Zucchini
- **Dinner:** Spaghetti Squash Bolognese
- **Dessert/Snack:** Tzatziki dip with baby carrot
- **Beverage:** Mango Mint Iced Green Tea

Day 21:

- **Breakfast:** Cheerios and Almond Milk Bowl
- **Lunch:** Spice Rub Grilled Tofu
- **Dinner:** Lebanese Kafta Kebabs with Tahini Sauce
- **Dessert/Snack:** Baked Bhakarwadi
- **Beverage:** Pomegranate Juice

Day 22:

- **Breakfast:** Chia seeds pudding with berries and coconut flakes
- **Lunch:** Chicken and Vegetable Wrap with Ginger Sauce
- **Dinner:** Herb-Infused Quinoa Medley
- **Dessert/Snack:** Chocolate Fudge Pie
- **Beverage:** Beetroot Juice

Day 23:

- **Breakfast:** Viking Crispbread with salmon
- **Lunch:** Tuna Salad Stuffed Tomato with Whole Grain Crackers
- **Dinner:** Eggplant & Lentil Bake
- **Dessert/Snack:** Peanut Butter Cookies
- **Beverage:** Pu-erh tea

Day 24:

- **Breakfast:** Walnut or Pecan Apple Oatmeal
- **Lunch:** Sweet Potato and Black Bean Tacos
- **Dinner:** Turkey Burger Bowl Salad

- **Dessert/Snack:** Baked Bhakarwadi

- **Beverage:** Mango Mint Iced Green Tea

Day 25:

- **Breakfast:** Blueberry and Granola Yogurt Parfait

- **Lunch:** Mushroom and Spinach Quesadillas

- **Dinner:** Green Goddess Supper

- **Dessert/Snack:** Tzatziki dip with baby carrot

- **Beverage:** Pomegranate Juice

Day 26:

- **Breakfast:** Toast with avocados and ricotta

- **Lunch:** Detox Roasted Pumpkin Soup

- **Dinner:** Barley-Stuffed Poblanos/Peppers

- **Dessert/Snack:** Celery sticks with hummus

- **Beverage:** Peach Smoothie

Day 27:

- **Breakfast:** Cheese and Veggie Egg White Breakfast Sandwich

- **Lunch:** Lemon Parsley Grilled Zucchini

- **Dinner:** Spaghetti Squash Bolognese

- **Dessert/Snack:** Chocolate Fudge Pie
- **Beverage:** Beetroot Juice

Day 28:

- **Breakfast:** Cheerios and Almond Milk Bowl
- **Lunch:** Spice Rub Grilled Tofu
- **Dinner:** Lebanese Kafta Kebabs with Tahini Sauce
- **Dessert/Snack:** Peanut Butter Cookies
- **Beverage:** Pu-erh tea

Day 29:

- **Breakfast:** Chia seeds pudding with berries and coconut flakes
- **Lunch:** Chicken and Vegetable Wrap with Ginger Sauce
- **Dinner:** Herb-Infused Quinoa Medley
- **Dessert/Snack:** Tzatziki dip with baby carrot
- **Beverage:** Mango Mint Iced Green Tea

Day 30:

- **Breakfast:** Viking Crispbread with salmon
- **Lunch:** Tuna Salad Stuffed Tomato with Whole Grain Crackers
- **Dinner:** Eggplant & Lentil Bake
- **Dessert/Snack:** Baked Bhakarwadi
- **Beverage:** Pomegranate Juice

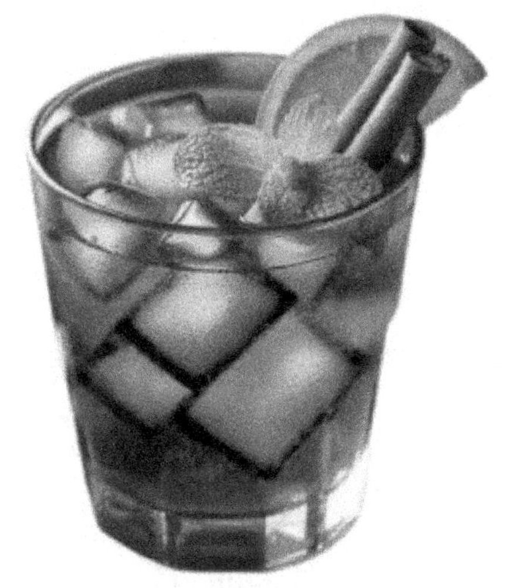

CHAPTER 4

Conclusion

Embarking on the journey of embracing a Fatty Liver Diet can be transformative, empowering, and ultimately life-changing for you.

Throughout this cookbook, you've discovered a wealth of delicious and nutritious recipes tailored specifically to support your liver health and overall well-being.

As you close the pages of this cookbook, remember that you hold the power to nourish your body and take control of your health.

Each recipe you've encountered here is not just a meal, but a step towards a healthier lifestyle.

From vibrant breakfast options to satisfying lunches, hearty dinners, and tantalizing desserts and snacks, you've explored a diverse array of culinary delights that prove eating for your liver can also be a pleasure for your palate.

But beyond the recipes lies a deeper message: a reminder that self-care is not selfish, but essential.

By choosing to prioritize your health and make mindful food choices, you're investing in a brighter, healthier future for yourself. It's about finding balance, enjoying delicious food, and feeling good from the inside out.

So, as you step into your kitchen armed with newfound knowledge and culinary inspiration, remember that you're not alone on this journey.

Whether you're cooking for yourself, your family, or friends, know that every meal you prepare is an act of self-love and nourishment.

As you savor each bite of these nutrient-packed meals, may you feel a renewed sense of vitality and well-being wash over you.

And as you continue on your path towards optimal health, may this cookbook serve as a trusted companion, guiding you towards a happier, healthier, and more vibrant life.

In the end, remember that the power to transform your health lies within you. With each meal you prepare, you're taking a step towards a healthier, happier you.

So, embrace the journey, savor the flavors, and nourish your body, mind, and spirit with every delicious bite.

With each mindful choice you make, you're one step closer to a life filled with wellness, joy, and abundance.

I appreciate the opportunity to be part of your journey. May your kitchen be filled with love, laughter, and the delicious aroma of nourishing meals for years to come. Here's to your health, happiness, and a future filled with culinary delights.